Mental Survival

Oliver Swingler

chipmunkapublishing
the mental health publisher

Oliver Swingler

All rights reserved, no part of this publication may be reproduced by any means, electronic, mechanical photocopying, documentary, film or in any other format without prior written permission of the publisher.

Published by
Chipmunkapublishing
United Kingdom

http://www.chipmunkapublishing.com

Copyright © 2016 *Oliver Swingler*
ISBN   978-1-78382-294-2

Mental health biopsy

I was first sent to a psychiatrist aged 13 in 1961, the Tavistock Clinic
Then in 1971 I was sectioned by my mother and sister, and in the short-stay Halliwick Hospital, diagnosed catatonic depressive and give ECT.

In 1974 I had a serious suicide attempt, recovery then 9 months in a Richmond Fellowship halfway house

I was registered with Newcastle mental health services in the late 1990, but got needed counselling via my GP and elsewhere

Oliver Swingler

Turning traumatic experience around

I once read that in ancient Amerindians tribes, if someone wanted to become a shaman – the healer and wise person – the first question asked was 'Have you ever experienced a major life crisis?' – and if the answer came 'No', they were not even accepted for training, as knowing life's traumas first-hand was considered an essential requirement for the empathy and understanding for the job.

Surviving PTSD, 'mental illness', does not necessarily bring wisdom, but it can offer a unique view, of both the human condition and society's ills. Depression and doubt, being forced inwards, and finding that accepted knowledge cannot adequately explain what is going on, can lead to a deepening and lifelong study, beginning with basic questions like 'Who am I?', 'What am I?', 'What does it mean to be human?' – and the painful, inspiring journey of thinking for oneself, challenging the mental strait-jacket of exam-laden school and college curricula.

In UK surveys of employers asked to rank who they would prefer not to take on from people who were women, black, old, LGBT, physically disabled, learning difficulty, ex-offender, mentally ill – we invariably come well last.

However, because of not despite the experience of stigmatisation, being considered amongst the lowest of the low, sometimes shunned by friends

Mental Survival

and foe alike, may potentially carry a defiant resilience bouncing back from rock bottom, and a stunning sensitivity and beautiful and caring empathy for the pain of others, and also by stripping away the false veneer of a civilised society – the greed and hypocrisy, cruelty and corruption – it can offer from the fringes a unique, insightful perspective of all that is wrong with the human community, and perhaps even ways to heal it, which the world ignores at its peril.

Oliver Swingler

Mental Health and GPs – letter to Healthwatch
19th June 2016
Dear Healthwatch,
I recently attended a meeting of Healthwatch in Newcastle, and as a result wrote the article below (copy sent to Healthwatch UK, and posted on various mental health Facebook sites).
If you get in touch with your local mental health groups, you may find they have similar experiences.

Best wishes,
Oliver Swingler

Ways in which mental health stigma can impact on physical health

It can be essential to get a mental diagnosis in order to access
support services such as counselling, or respite from employment whilst working through a traumatic episode, without facing dire poverty. However a diagnosis may then significantly affect a patient's physical health condition, in a number of ways.

Firstly, there's the attitude of doctors, many of whom are at least as ready to stigmatise as the general public. Because of having been fairly itinerant over the years, I've had many experiences of signing on with new surgeries. At the first visit I've usually get on well with the doctor – at college I knew a number of medical students, and I've worked in the NHS, so I can talk their language – and I'd have no trouble explaining my current symptoms and getting a prescription. But if I returned a few weeks later – in the meantime my medical records including mental health history having arrived – what met me would be totally different. The doctor would not look me in the eye, he'd talk loudly over me as if I were stupid, my described symptoms such as where I felt pain would not be believed, and I'd sometimes go away without any medication, feeling a lot worse for my visit.

At a recent local HealthWatch meeting, a carer described how his daughter, who was diagnosed as bipolar, was assigned to a particular doctor in the practice – and however bad her physical health, no other doctor would see her, and the next appointment might be a month away. By which time her untreated physical health condition might have got a whole lot worse.

On one occasion she urgently needed attention, and had to really shout loudly before anyone listened. Having had a similar experience, I then chipped in that a further problem could arise – the doctor might write into medical record that "the patient was aggressive" (no I/she wasn't, we were ill and extremely upset at not being believed!) as a permanent record, and any future doctor would be even less likely to be sympathetic.

Another patient described how he was having real, painful and even life threatening problems with his pace-maker – but was not believed by a number of health professionals – and having only fairly recently had a mental health episode, he was able to differentiate between the attitude of staff before and after he was known as being a mental health survivor. Eventually after weeks of unnecessary pain, they did decide to investigate, which took a minute or two, a very simple mistake had been made, and the problem rectified in a few seconds. But in a sense he was fortunate, some mental health survivors are never believed, until a bit too late, after the autopsy,

Then there's the problem of time. A patient may go to the GP needing some help with mental health problems as well as one or more physical health conditions. Physical symptoms are hard enough to describe, mental health problems even more so, and the allotted 10 minutes per appointment can easily not be sufficient. I've had the experience of being told that my time was up, and I hadn't even mentioned two physical health problems, which therefore got no treatment until I could make a further appointment a week or more away.

I'm sure many mental health survivors have their own stories of receiving below standard care of physical health at the hands of their GP. And the appalling fact is that the death rate of mental health survivors is significantly higher than the average, even if suicide is factored out.

We shouldn't and needn't put up with it, and as a first step I would urge everyone with a personal experience of poor care to contact your local Healthwatch, and pass it on, so they can collate experiences, and take it up with higher authorities

Mental Survival

within the NHS and government. And maybe one day medical professionals will treat us with the dignity and respect we deserve, and sometimes so urgently need.

Best wishes,
Oliver Swingler

Oliver Swingler

Suggestions for dealing with the DWP etc:

If possible, whenever going for an assessment, take a witness – perhaps a solicitor (though no longer legal aid), or an advocate (though most advocacy projects have suffered funding cuts), perhaps a member of a union, community or faith group, or a friend or member of your family ..

And/or if possible record the whole assessment – I'm a mental
health survivor with memory problems, and I used to proclaim my right to record – which they didn't like but gave way. Better openly – because my experience is their behaviour will be far more respectful. But if not, perhaps you or your witnesses do it surreptitiously – then at least you can challenge any subsequent lies they might weave.

When sending e-mails (or letters) to the DWP, or Maximus, Capita etc, ALWAYS put Cc at the bottom, and copy it to your local MP and local councillor (both of whom have been elected to protect your lawful rights), and/or advocacy project, community group etc. I now usually get a thank you from at least one councillor, asking to be kept informed, and the implied threat that you won't take unjust decisions lying down can work wonders for their sense of public service (if any!).

Over the years of having multiple dealings with various bodies, as a result of having both physical disability and mental health problems, and more than 30 jobs and periods of unemployment in-

Mental Survival

between – I became fairly well-known as an assertive citizen (or perhaps 'trouble-maker'?!) – and after making a number of complaints, always with help and support (and winning compensation from tribunals) – I eventually tended to get a much quicker response, and my full entitlement with few problems.

More suggestions for assessments:
Prepare your case – don't just try to ad-lib – make copious notes of all your symptoms in detail, take all the back-up documents you've got, from your doctor, hospital, social worker, carer – and make sure they have copies (you might even ask for a receipt?!). And if your evidence doesn't fit within any of their questions – especially if you've got a witness and/or are recording the interview on you mobile – make sure you say it anyway – and ask loudly after each point "Have you made a note of that?" – and repeat it if they refuse to say 'Yes'!

In social situations, when asked 'How are you?', people often reply 'I'm fine, how are you?' even when they are not. When going to an assessment –before you even walk through the door of the building, let alone the interview room, you need to brace yourself to DO THE OPPOSITE! If you've got a condition which is in any way variable – and we all have good and bad days – make sure ALL your answers are from the point of view of when you are AT YOUR WORST. For instance, two of my chronic conditions are psoriatic arthritis and depression, both of which are variable. So if asked, can I walk 50 metres (or whatever it is now) I'd absolutely honestly say something like

Oliver Swingler

"On a bad day – which is on average about 4 days a week – I have trouble getting out of bed, and definitely can't leave the flat, so no I can't". (I would not say, "On a good day, I can go into town, and with my walking-stick and a couple of pauses walk down the High Street" – even though that was also true). I never lied – but however nice and sympathetic best buddies they pretended to be, I would insist on detailing and even acting out (sometimes with a.bit of drama!) my very real disturbed thoughts and memories, physical aches and pains. (I only learnt I had to do that having once been stuck in my flat, my two best friends away on holiday, with very little money and food for about 10 days!).

Mental Survival

Counselling experiences in the UK

Some years ago I'd reached a crisis point, desperately needing counselling, or more precisely talking therapy.   I was broke, but managed to get the local Mental Health Trust to fund some sessions (they knew me as a serial complainer/agitator who wouldn't go away!).

They sent a list of 'approved counsellors' and I wrote to half a dozen – who all turned me down – too complex issues, didn't deal with mental health survivors (!?!), other spurious reasons.

So I went through my GP – who could only offer students who knew far less than I did about what they were supposed to be doing (I almost ended up running master classes!) – which wasn't much good for my needs!   And it was only one hour a week, far too little – so simultaneously I went to the addiction agency for free sessions, and managed to barter more with a holistic healer – I just needed to talk.

Eventually I came across a group called Someone Cares which offered counselling for people 'affected by sexual abuse' (I was physically, emotionally, mentally bullied as a child –but not sexually – though I'd discovered that both my parents had suffered childhood sexual abuse, and was beginning to think their horrific experience the root cause of my issues).   And there were three things different – firstly, I'm physically disabled, and she was prepared to come to my flat (whilst her partner waited outside until she let him know she felt safe with me).

Secondly, she herself had been abused as a child, a lovely woman with a tremendous store of empathy who immediately knew exactly what I was talking about, which was so incredibly refreshing.

And thirdly, there was no clock watching – the 1st session lasted about 2 and a half hours until I'd talked myself out, the 2nd just over an hour. After which I didn't feel I needed any more – my immediate desperation to talk and make sense of things was satisfied, I'd lots to think about in my own time, emergency over – and all the after-effects were positive!

Now I'm not saying this would've suited everybody –we all have different needs at different times – but it struck me that although cash-starved Mental Health Trusts may favour the 'quick fix' of psycho-drugs and ECT (and then the chronic after-effects which may last a lifetime), my two session were much more cost-effective.

I'm not advocating more flexible talking therapies just on the grounds that they're cheaper – there are far more important reasons for investing in them. But in today's world, money talks – and perhaps we sometimes need to sink to the level of the consultants, accountants and bureaucrats to show that it's yet another reason for replacing the psychiatrists' option – although of course if they're getting lots of freebies from ten different drug companies and ECT manufacturers, all-expenses-paid ''conferences'' in the Seychelles, it might fall on deaf ears.

Oliver Swingler

Four encounters with UK psychiatrists

Firstly I was sent to a clinic having naughtily aged 12/13 been bunking off school, stealing, parties etc. I was given some shadow drawing and asked to make up a story, and having a vivid imagination, I was happy to oblige. What I hadn't realised till later was they were going to use my story to analyse me – they could have but hadn't told me that – which I regarded as utterly deceitful – and have distrusted and refused co-operation with psychiatrists ever since.

The main "analysis" (likely the same whatever my story had been!) was 'you're jealous of your father and want to have sex with your mother' which was a totally new idea to me and not easy for an early adolescent boy to cope with. (What made it particularly outrageous is that I discovered when 39 (the first person my mother ever told) that both my parents had been raped when they were children, my working-class mother by her first-world-war traumatised veteran father, my middle-class father at his public school).

Then some months later, my usual psychiatrist was away, and I saw another, getting the second wonderful insight: 'You have strong homosexual tendencies and fancy the first psychiatrist'. Which I thought hilarious because even at primary school I'd earned a reputation for constantly chasing after girls! I worked out that it was a classic case of transference (i.e I actually really didn't like him, but was aware that he fancied me, but homosexuality – let alone paedophilia – was illegal in those days, and he couldn't cope with that fact!) when he had a 'breakdown', which I was lead to believe was in large part my fault! And this was at the world-renowned Tavistock Clinic (now I believe the Tavistock Institute of Human Relations).

Third encounter, whilst exhausted and grieving the death of my father, I was sectioned by my mother and sister, given deep sleep therapy, and then when I didn't get 'well' quickly enough – it was a short-stay hospital – given ECT. As far as I can recollect, and it is hazy, the psychiatrist saw me for about 5 minutes and didn't ask me a single direct question. Some weeks later I wanted out from the clinic, and another patient suggested going to art therapy, and painting a picture using only bright colours signifying I was getting better, dark equalling depression! And it worked, the art therapist got very excited, this time I did have a conversation with the psychiatrist, lied through my teeth about how positive I felt, and was set free.

On the fourth occasion, I was lying in a hospital bed, bandages on both wrists, my stomach pumped (a long story, another time!), when a psychiatrist walked in, sat on the end of the bed, and spread notes about me around so that they were visible to me. About all he said was 'What are we going to do with you?' – This was different, he actually wanted my opinion; back in 1974, this was revolutionary!

At University, I'd a friend studying psychology, who'd then got a job with the Richmond Fellowship – so that's what I suggested. And the

psychiatrist got me an interview, for which I'm very grateful, and I was in a half-way house for 9 months.
But the thing is, he didn't need umpteen year training to do what he did, just to be a decent human being with some empathy. I suspect that the training actually erodes what empathy medical students have (though things might have changed) , and he was jut someone who'd slipped through the professional net.

Mental Survival

Sexual assault by professionals

Here's another hot topic which may or may not have come up before.

Back in late 90s/early 2000s I was a member then Chair of Lifeboat, Tyneside Mental Health Co-operative, which was a totally self-running mental health survivors support group, no professionals involved whatsoever.

One day we were discussing professional abuse, and took a straw poll, and as far as I can remember, all the women members, and about half the men had experienced sexual harassment – varying from inappropriate touching or groping, to rape – at the hands of a doctor or psychiatrist who was supposedly treating them.

There was a common theme that if they made any sort of suggestion of complaining, they were threatened that they would no longer be prescribed psychiatric drugs they'd become addicted to, they'd be blacklisted so have extreme difficulty finding another doctor, and told anyway, who would believe someone who was certified 'mad, crazy' etc against the word of a respected pillar of the community.
Just as the Savile revelations have proved to be the tip of the iceberg, I suspect that the sexual abuse of mental health survivors has a long history and still goes on in hospitals and surgeries around the country – it's the ultimate power trip for corrupt psychiatrists.

Oliver Swingler

It's not something I've experienced myself – but hearing the poignant stories of some lovely, vulnerable people taken advantage of and unable to fight back made me extremely angry – and maybe at some point a class action, public enquiry could happen –and perhaps if someone wants to take it on board, to start with the collection of people's stories (with names, dates, places if possible, but anonymously if preferred) – however long ago – which may not be able to be proven, but if there are lots of them, it could be enough to get a human rights organisation or MP interested (which is something I'm good at).

Mental Survival

Direct Action!

What really happens when people take direct action? Oliver Swingler sent us is experience (see article below) showing it's not always as negative as some people think:

To the Chairperson
Newcastle City Health NHS Trust
I am writing to let you know that on Tuesday 3rd April (2000) at 11am, it is my intention to stand outside the Hadrian Clinic, giving out an information sheet entitled '48 facts you need to know before agreeing to ECT'. Please note that I am not asking your permission, I am simply informing you of my intention. ...

I am taking this action in support of the Secretary of State for Health's recent statement that 'informed consent of patients and families is paramount'. I strongly believe from my own experience, confirmed by extensive surveys (by ECT Anonymous, UKAN and MIND), that mental health patients are being given ECT without full information and without consent, and that it causes long-term damage to both physical and mental health. My MP, Jim Cousins, has written saying he is taking up the matter of informed consent with the Government on my behalf – but it could take years to effect change, and in the meanwhile, vulnerable people are being harmed. I also have very personal reason. Like over 60% of ECT survivors, I suffer from a fear of doctors and hospitals, and have for 30 years. This fear was exacerbated on Tuesday, when I was

approached, on your instructions, by two large security guards and intimidated into hobbling quickly from the hospital premises. Rather than giving way to my fear, I have decided to face it, as a step towards overcoming the victim mentality that ECT helped induce in me, and a way of empowering myself – empowerment of mental health survivors being a principle that the Health Trust says it considers important ...
Oliver Swingler

What Happened Next! ECT Action Day April 3rd
WE arrived at the Hadrian Clinic, Newcastle General Hospital, expecting to be asked to leave immediately (as 2 weeks ago) – but, lo and behold, a victory! Since April 1st Newcastle, Notrt Tyneside and Northumberland Health Trusts have merged, and instead of two burly security guards, the brand new Communications Officer greeted us. She was very charming and reasonable – she admitted they'd totally over-reacted before, and had no problem with us being there and handing out the 48 point fact sheet on ECT (lucky I'd brought some!).

And it was worth it! Besides giving them out to patients and staff, we met two visitors. The first was a man visiting his wife, who'd been hospitalised suffering from post-natal depression. He said she'd been getting on OK before ECT, but then had lost it, all over the place, couldn't remember things, and even handle being in the kitchen – it had really changed her, and he was really worried.

Mental Survival

The second was a mother whose now only child, a woman of 50 was hospitalised suffering from grief after her only sister had died. The mother was terrified that through ECT she'd lose her only daughter. She said she wanted to move her to a private hospital – but I warned her that they had an ECT clinic there also.

I gave them contact information, recommended the Advocacy Centre, and a solicitor who deals in mental health and promised to help all I could.

I feel totally drained – from wondering what might happen (last night visions of being arrested or sectioned) and then the two traumatic conversations, But I'll be back – maybe a regular weekly visit – and I'll keep you informed.

Wow – this is real empowerment!
Oliver Swingler –Tyneside ECT Anonymous (TEA for short – it's better for you, and a whole lot safer than ECT)
Published in The Advocate May 2001

Oliver Swingler

Here's my ECT story, after only a few shocks, written in 2000

ECT after-effects – a survivor's story

What I didn't know until I was 39 is that I was brought up in a family affected by sexual abuse, both my parents had suffered childhood rape, and being the youngest I bore the brunt of sibling bullying, a 'juvenile delinquent' survivor of psychiatry from 1961 getting the usual Freudian 'you're jealous of your father and want to have sex with your mother' plus told that I had strong homosexual tendencies, and fancied my first psychiatrist – I was 12 at the time – a classic case of transference – all of which made me uncooperative with psychiatrists – a big mistake!!

In 1971 I was in a grieving process and exhausted from running a summer play scheme, so they sectioned me, diagnosed catatonic depression, filled me up to the eyeballs with drugs, and when I didn't 'get better' quick enough, without any choice or mention of the after-effects, they gave me ECT – I don't know how many shocks, or whether, as is common practice, the equipment was obsolete, the staff untrained, the voltage totally arbitrary, because, it seems, when I started to make noises about suing, they conveniently lost my medical records.

Soon after ECT, I was visited in hospital by someone whose face and name I didn't know, although, I learnt in conversation we'd shared a communal flat, eating drinking, talking together almost every day of the previous year, and when I was despatched back with no after-care to the family home where problems had arisen, I discovered my current address book, and frantically phoned some strange names in it, hoping their voices would bring back glimmers of recognition.

Soon after ECT I realised I could remember all of the alphabet, nor my times table although I'd As in maths GCE O and A level, and I often stayed at home, irrationally fearing I'd be asked to recite them – for weeks I didn't know first names of my parents, older siblings – at the first opportunity I moved to a town where almost no-one knew me, to avoid the embarrassment of social situations, and I still have cold sweats in large groups when I might be called upon to introduce people I'd known for years, but can't remember their names – every day I need to muster the courage to venture forth so as not to be trapped in lonely isolation.

For 6 or so years after my finals, sat just before ECT, I thought I'd failed, until writing about something else, with a vague ps, I was sent my degree certificate, which was useful, no longer having to explain away 4 years of my life – I've got 13 GCEs, 4 top grade, but no professional qualifications – since ECT I've sat only 1 exam, and despite it being 70% project work and continual assessment, I struggled to just pass, well bottom of the class – my memory and impaired concentration can't cope.

Oliver Swingler

Some years after ECT, I was approached by a Social Security inspector, who asked if I knew a woman, and was surprised when I didn't, but insisted she was the mother of my daughter – having no memory of her, I was easily persuaded by my now ex-wife to deny paternity – years later again, I met old friends, who said I'd had an affair, and she'd just had her womb scraped – but by then I'd thrown away all the papers, and am told I can't now trace her, and she's unlikely to want to trace me, who forgot being her father.

I can spend all afternoon in deep, personal conversation with one other person, then, the very next day in the street cut her or him dead, walk away from the smile of, to me, a total stranger, which has lost me untold friends (I didn't know I did that until a kind person told me), and I've long since given up on my life aim of writing a novel – my mind can only extend to brief, disciplined sections (like this is written) – even though at college my published articles got a special mention in an award-winning Observer Mace student magazine.

For 29 years I've lived a moment to moment existence, every day coping with an emotional yo-yo – I'm liable to cry in company for no apparent reason, leaving my flat is a major expedition, and I rarely go beyond a round of known people and places, partly because explaining to those who don't know me why I reacted in a particular way is just too complicated, and for a long time my sleep was rare – like those twitching frog's legs, I suffer from muscular spasms that jerk me awake when I lie down and try to relax.

Like many ECT survivors, I suffer from fear of doctors and hospitals, and a few years ago I had uveitis, but kept putting off seeing my doctor, until two friends almost dragged me there, and then to hospital, where I was told, another week and there'd have been permanent damage and blindness – I've had at least three 'mystery' illnesses, and perhaps like others a brain scan would show the same results as a stroke or epileptic fit caused by ECT – but they are serious medical conditions, whilst ECT is supposed to be a treatment.

I'm told ECT is given to cure suicidal tendencies, which I find very peculiar, because before ECT I was never suicidal, and when a friend killed himself, I was horrified by the waste of life and talent – but 3 years after ECT I almost did it, countless crushed up pills and my wrists still bear the scars, and every week, almost every day, my thoughts turn to suicide, my urge to live is weak, dormant – and it's odd that if ECT is such a life-saver, why is the death rate for those who've had it so much higher than the national average?

Childhood family holidays were all over Europe, I did a year's VSO abroad, then hitchhiked across South Africa, and when at college in 1968 from Rome to Copenhagen and home, but since ECT I haven't ventured outside the UK, I'm not sure I could manage – after ECT and the suicide attempt it helped induce, I spent a year in a halfway house, but then, realising I couldn't cope alone, I was easy meat for recruitment to a group I fooled myself into believing was honourable, learning 19 years later it was a cult with a guru motivated by greed – where had gone the independent free spirit I once was?

ECT is given by professionals who admit they don't know what it does, except to say it's localised brain treatment, yet the human body is 70% or more water, an excellent conductor, so how can they guarantee it's just local – in a recent survey of ECT survivors, over a third said it had damage them, so every day doctors are breaking their Hippocratic Oath 'do no harm' – to me ECT equals Every Cell Traumatised, I've been tortured in civilised fashion, and all the time have to struggle against the victim mentality it's helped produce in me.

At a recent kinesiology session, I was taken through the experience of having ECT, to help heal it, and whilst she gently held my hand, it was as if I was ejected into the air, and I was left with the feeling of pure, unadulterated TERROR – I don't own a TV, it affects me too much, and go to the cinema about once a year – Schindler's List left me shattered for about a month, and Jurassic Park gave me nightmares and daymares for weeks, as if ECT had punched a hole in my aura, destroyed protection from outside influences.

But I've been lucky, unlike the hundreds who die during treatment, written off as 'heart attack', or are paralysed, or have given up, their minds

Mental Survival

destroyed, or are forced to agree to yet more shocks under threat of denial of psychiatric drugs they've been made addicts of – an American philosopher once wrote 'Those who cannot remember the past are condemned to repeat it', and I've spent weeks vainly trying to recall lost months, but can't fill the gaps – I often feel I'm going round in circles, and about all that keeps me going is anger at what was done to me.

Oliver Swingler
Written 28th October 2000 – slightly edited September 2015

And later …

Since writing and sharing my ECT survivors story, I got lots of support from others who'd been damaged by the mental health system, got out some of my anger manning a picket outside an ECT clinic (my picture was in the local newspaper!), had loads of counselling – about my dysfunctional family affected by sexual abuse, leaving the cult, near alcoholism and being an ex-offender, as well as psychiatric and ECT abuse. And, in the course of a year, I tried 20 different forms of alternative therapy – using barter for those I couldn't afford, and even found a sympathetic doctor who actually listened.

I still live moment-to-moment and have memory problems – but people pay big bucks to learn to live in now, when I can't do anything else (!), and I've pieced together much of my life story, important names and dates, which is always nearby in case of panic attacks.

My anti-ECT stance helped me regain some of the campaigning zeal of my youth, and I've broadened out, been involved in anti-war and anti-fracking protests, as well as for a time joining a left/green choir, and writing two songs: 'Bees are buzzing' https://youtu.be/TwHZkY4Ubfl and 'Global warming' http://youtu.be/s9g_Ucr4twQ both of which have been retweeted by hundreds of people to more than a million followers.

I still have problems in social situations, but I've two very good friends, have served on a committee or two, and even had the confidence to get back onto the dating scene, chatting away to others seeking friendship.

What I'm trying to get across is that it's not easy, but it isn't all bad news, there can be life after ECT, moments of joy as well as sorrow, and with my sights and expectations of myself set nice and low, the chance to have real self-respect knowing I tried, I did something I feel good about almost every day.

Best wishes,
Oliver
14th September 2015

Mental Survival

In my 40 years as an ECT survivor, I've yet to meet a single person who gave informed consent –as the Royal College of Psychiatrists ECT Handbook requires.

This is a fact-sheet compiled in 2000 , and handed out during a picket I did of the Hadrian ECT clinic in Newcastle – I was escorted off the hospital grounds by some large porters, but was invited to return the next day after I'd been interviewed ion local radio, and my picture and short article in the Newcastle Chronicle.

You are welcome to amend, update, pick and choose from the fact-sheet for any similar demos ...

48 facts you need to know before agreeing to ECT

1. Early pioneers of medicine used to test their cures on themselves, but no longer – an American ECT survivor has offered $5,000 on the Internet to any doctor willing to undergo 10 shock treatments (the usual course), but there have been no takers.
2. Every doctor used to take the Hippocratic Oath, which says "Do no harm" – but in a UKAN survey of ECT survivors more than 35% said it had damaged them.
3. The [UK] Royal College of Psychiatrist (RCP) 1996 audit reported that 67% of clinics were not following the guidelines on safety in giving ECT.

4. On Women's Hour [a very popular BBC4 radio programme] in January 2000 a clinical psychiatrist told of interviewing patients, who described the process of being given ECT as "feeling assaulted, punished, humiliated, stigmatised; they felt betrayed and degraded and worthless, and there was an overall feeling of having been helpless and out of control".

5. A pro-ECT American psychiatrist has written: "The objectives of electro-shock therapy is to produce ... a condition of confusion which we term 'complete depatterning'" – in other words, brain-washing.

6. ECT survivors in this country (UK) have experienced the following physical after-effects: muscle spasms, palpitations, back pain, muscle pain, joint pain, bowel problems, thyroid problems, stress ulcers, undiagnosed nervous system condition, dehydration – and lots more.

7. In an ECT Anonymous survey, over 50% experienced the after-effects of impaired number skills, impaired language/writing, panic attacks, bad dreams or nightmares, suicidal tendencies.

8. Two doctors, working in Italy when it was ruled by Fascism, are hailed as being the pioneers of ECT experiments on human beings.

9. A report on ECT stated that it produces a temporary feeling of well-being and

Mental Survival

permanent harm to memory, similar to strokes, asphyxiation, concussion, carbon monoxide poisoning – but they are serious medical conditions, whilst ECT is supposed to be a cure.

10 The [UK] Secretary of State for Health recently said: "Informed consent of patients and families is paramount" – but the RCP Handbook states that "In some cases ECT is necessary even if the patient refuses consent."

11 Under ECT, increased doses of electricity are given to produce a fit – yet neurologists work hard to reduce fits in people suffering from epilepsy at all costs, knowing that fits can produce permanent brain damage.

12 The [UK] 1998 Benbow Report stated that 25% of psychiatrists had seen a "death or major medical complication" on the ECT table.

13 In Victorian times, a black box giving electric shocks was advertised as a good way of dealing with 'wayward wives and difficult servants' – from January to March 1999, of 2,800 patients in the UK given ECT, over two-thirds were women.

14 After more than 60 years of using it, psychiatrists admit that they do not understand how ECT works – but deny that they are experimenting.

15 A 1998 report found that 64% of consultant psychiatrists had not even

read the RCP Handbook giving guidelines on ECT safety.

16. Here is a typical experience of memory loss from an ECT survivor: "Patients come up to me and say 'Hi'. They know me, but I have no idea who they are. They don't even look familiar. They say I spent a long time with them, but I have no memory. Part of me is missing forever".

17. An American Psychiatric Association report states that: "In many patients, the recovery from retrograde amnesia will be incomplete, and there is evidence that ECT can result in persistent or permanent memory loss."

18. A pro-ECT psychiatrist recently agreed that working through traumatic childhood events can be vital for long-term settlement of a mental health problem – but that becomes impossible if ECT has destroyed accurate memory of them.

19. In an ECT Anonymous survey, over 60% of ECT survivors said they had the after-effects of impaired organisational skills, feeling of remoteness, personality changes, fear of doctors and hospitals.

20. Major advances in pioneering ECT research took place in Nazi Germany, where doctors and psychiatrists had thousands of concentration camp victims to experiment on, and death on the ECT table saved the cost of transport to the gas chamber.

Mental Survival

21 A 1985 ECT researcher stated: "There is not a single methodologically sound study that reports beneficial effects lasting as long as four weeks."

22 Here are some comments overheard from therapists giving ECT … "Let's give him the works" … "Hit him with all we've got" … "The patient was noisy and restive, so I put him on intensive ECT three times a day" … " .. a mental spanking .. ".

23 ECT treatment aims to approach the threshold dose of electricity – shocks higher than the threshold will cause 'cognitive impairment in proportion to the overshock' – 'This threshold dose varies 1 to 40 from one patient to another' – 'Clinics have no way of determining the threshold dose' – ' … routine settings vary fourfold between clinics'.

24 Psychiatrists say that ECT is a life-saver when people are suicidal – but a 1999 Journal of Clinical Psychiatrists article states that: "Proof remains elusive that any medical intervention has produced a measurable impact on suicide rates in the general population".

25 Here are some anagrams of "Electro-convulsive therapy": Volt virulence rapes the coy …Convey torture vehicle slap … Every volt lot is pure chance … Cruelly not revive past echo … Ever cancel host love purity … The lovely nature crops vice …

26 Some psychiatrists describe ECT as 'a treatment of last resort', others say it is 'a preferred treatment', still others have written that it is 'cruel and barbaric', that it should be banned, and that effective humane alternative techniques do exist.

27 Recently a woman referred by a Rape Crisis Centre was told by a psychiatrist, after 30 minutes conversation, that he could diagnose her as schizophrenic or manic depressive or personality disorder – some psychiatrists will prescribe ECT for all these labels, some for none.

28 Here are some comments from ECT survivors after treatment ... "Why do I feel like a robot?" ... "Why am I so fatigued all the time?" ... "Why can't I remember day-to-day things like I used to?' ... "Are others so scared a I am of visiting the doctor?"

29 EEG tests have shown that ECT dramatically affects theta and delta rhythms of the brain, indicating brain deterioration and damage.

30 ECT survivors who have had a brain scan have been asked "Are you epileptic or have you had a stroke?" – the technician was puzzled when they said no, but when they revealed that they'd had ECT, said "That explains it!"

31 In the ECT Anonymous survey of survivors, 76% said they were unable to return to their previous occupation (and a further 17% only partially), whilst 70%

could not even take up less demanding work – not a very good record for a supposed cure.

32 During the Second World War, exhausted and traumatised Nazi soldiers returning from the Russian front, who refused to fight any more, were given ECT to erase their memory of the horror, then sent back, often to their death.

33 Some patients who swear by ECT were not told they were taking part in a research experiment, and were in a 'no treatment' control group – so maybe being put to sleep under anaesthetic is a better option, with fewer risks and damaging side-effects.

34 An ECT Anonymous survey did not show much 'informed consent' – 86% of ECT survivors felt they had been pressurised into having ECT, whilst 96% felt that the risks had not been properly explained to them.

35 An American philosopher, George Santayana, has written: "Those who cannot remember the past are condemned to repeat it" – but ECT damages the memory.

36 A Nottingham study of ECT survivors found that those under 65 had a mortality rate of four times the national average and a greater risk of readmission to hospital, whilst results of a recent Scottish audit of ECT, of 1,314 patients receiving 8,672 treatments,

suggests that there is an ECT related death in Scotland every 3 days.

37 A man recently won £500,000 compensation after a 15-year legal battle, having been paralysed from the waist down on the ECT table.

38 A recent report on ECT in America showed that 92% of psychiatrists there don't prescribe it, and of the remaining 8% most were trained in the UK.

39 A consultant recently stated that psychiatrists receive no financial benefit from giving ECT – but the RCP Handbook extensively quotes from US research funded by major manufacturers of ECT equipment, research which of course 'proved' that ECT is completely safe and effective, and ECT equipment manufacturers are extremely generous in sponsoring all-expenses-paid 'conferences' in places like the Seychelles and Bahamas!

40 After receiving shock treatment, the writer Ernest Hemingway wrote: "What is the sense of ruining my head and erasing my memory, which is my capital, and putting me out of business? It was a brilliant cure but we lost the patient" – soon after, he killed himself.

41 Rorschach tests after ECT revealed: "The dullness which is characteristic, immediately following shock therapy, often persisted for a long time, in some cases years after shock" … "rigidity in the use of mental resources" …

"inattention and inability to concentrate" ... "difficulty in carrying out tasks that they were well trained to do before their illness".

42 Other tests have recorded the immediate after-effects of "confusion, headaches, disorientation, muscle ache, physical weakness, dizziness" ... and ..."memory loss, apathy (emotional blunting), learning difficulties, and loss of creativity, drive and energy may last for weeks, months, or even be permanent".

43 In the ECT Anonymous survey, over 80% survivors had experienced loss of past memory, impaired present memory, and impaired concentration.

44 Some psychiatric nurses and technicians have experienced horror and trauma from witnessing ECT being given – it is hoped that they then refused to administer it, rather than using the excuse "We were only following orders" (as they said at the Nuremberg trials).

45 ECT survivors will be pleased to learn that "The tendency for death to occur in ECT recipients earlier than non-recipients does not become pronounced until 5 or 10 years following first hospitalisation".

46 A 1996 survey showed that in the UK, 12 young people under 18 were given ECT, including a child of 12 – the ECT Handbook recommends that the option

47 be kept open for giving ECT to children even younger.

47 Modern 'modified' ECT is supposed to be safer, but because of the drugs and anaesthetic given, it actually utilises even more electricity than in the past, up to 450 volts, to produce an epileptic coma, just as happened before ECT was 'modified'.

48 An ECT survivor has written: "Just when I needed care and help, they damaged my brain … I was never suicidal before ECT, but 3 years later I nearly killed myself, needing life-support, and a year in a half-way house … 30 years later I still live day-to-day, I'm an emotional yo-yo .. about the only thing that keeps me going is anger about what was done to me, and thousands of other people .. if I can help to see it banned, my pain and torment will have been worthwhile …"

Fact sheet produced by Oliver Swingler in March 2000.

ECT Informed consent

Of the ECT survivors I've met, or who took part in a UK ECT Anonymous survey some years ago, a few have said were coerced into having the treatment. The majority remembered being given almost no information and didn't give consent (having not been asked!). A sizeable minority recall being given little or misinformation – such as "You might lose some memory for a few days, but it will all come back very quickly" – and gave consent. But I have yet to meet a single person who was told beforehand of the entire list of potential side-effects, and how likely they were – and then gave 'informed consent'.

In contrast, it's an absolute requirement that every packet of drugs sold in a UK chemist – paracetamol, aspirin, the lot – has a comprehensive list of side-effects, listed in order of severity, giving how likely they are. So that if you don't like them, you can decide not to take the tablets, and maybe ask the doctor for an alternative.

My vague, foggy and distant memory is that I was told to join a line of sitting patients, having not been given any information and certainly not giving consent. And unfortunately I'd been so drugged up for a week or so, suitably meek and compliant, that if they'd told me to scratch my head all day, I probably would have done it.

I can't prove that – I can't even prove I've had ECT as they've lost my medical records – but you can bet your life that if I had signed an 'Informed consent' form, they would have found that very quickly, especially when, almost 30 years later, I started muttering threats to sue.

If there are enough 'cases' confirmed by neurologists, it may then be possible to interest a human rights organisation to fund a pro-bono class action – but it'll have to be really substantial evidence. I suspect that only after a very high-profile court case – which the ECT manufacturers and professional bodies of psychiatrist will fight tooth-and-nail all the way – will there be a major policy shift – because in health care nowadays it's money not care that talks –and only the fear of substantial damage will get them to see sense.

I think we're a long way yet – but absolutely – collecting evidence with professional evidence of neurologists has got to be a first step.

Some years – like a few other ECT survivors over the years – I approached Amnesty to try to get them to recognise ECT without informed consent as torture – but although they could recognise that not all psychiatrists are good guys – eg use by Stalinist Russia to have a sectioned hundreds of dissidents –they wouldn't touch it, and communication ended acrimoniously – they basically still believe 'the exert'. But if we have tens of cases substantiated by another set of experts actually held in higher standing than psychiatrists amongst the medical profession (which neurologists certainly are, a re-approach to them, or Liberty etc, would be well worth while.

Mental Survival

ECT, memory and abuse

When I've been campaigning against ECT, I've been surprised that – despite all the evidence of lack of informed consent, of brain damage, of debilitating side-effects (catalogued by ECT Anonymous amongst others) – there hasn't been universal condemnation even amongst mental health survivors. And over the years I've even met a number of people who swear by it, and have struggled to understand why.

For me a major after-effect has been memory problems, chronic and on-going. Right after ECT, I realised I couldn't remember my 3 siblings and parents first names, recite the alphabet or my times table – and after having been highly literate, I had to do a series of exercise which involved scanning through a concise dictionary more than 100 times to have any hope of not frequently stopping mid-sentence in conversations, vainly searching my brain for a lost word. And i used to avoid social situation, lest I be caught out in some forgetfulness, and look a fool.

'Those who cannot remember the past are condemned to repeat it' (George Santayana) is one of my favourite sayings – and of course ECT doesn't help! Over the years on a number of occasions I've badgered, cajoled family, old friends making copious notes, looked in newspapers and contemporary diaries, constructed flow charts and timelines, asking 'what happened, what did I do, who said what, etc

etc???' It was an instinctive quest, and whole lot of hard work (some repeated when I forgot I'd done it before!) but I knew I had to do it, and even though I'm still not sure whether I've regained a memory, or built a fiction around someone else's partial and one-sided recollection, it's been worth it, to overcome the alienation of ECT, and regain some feeling of who I am, of being my own person.

For those who swear by ECT, my main conjecture is this, that for some people, memories of childhood – perhaps including child rape, physical and emotional abuse, unremitting bullying and belittling – are so utterly horrific, that even ifopen-ended talking therapy coupled with close PTSD support were available, the temporary relief (and it is temporary, suddenly intruding flashbacks can always recur) of memory loss is preferable. But I'd welcome any other theories, and I'm happy to debate respectfully with someone who thinks different.

There is one certainty, that ECT precludes any justice for victims of such childhood trauma. Victims who, however many years later, have mustered the enormous courage to pursue and confront their abuser in court, and obtained a conviction and fitting punishment, often express a degree of satisfaction, and the beginnings of coming to terms with what happened, and move on. But if someone has had ECT, it becomes impossible – any half-decent perpetrator's defence lawyer would tear to shreds evidence from an ECT survivor, who would have to admit to severe memory problems. So you could call ECT the 'cure' of choice of paedophiles for their victims.

Oliver Swingler

My muddled mind

My muddled mind lurches along the undercurrents
Of their persuasive words, desperately struggling to perceive
The hidden agendas, avoid the whirlpools of polluted expertise,
The brittle shells of their unconscious mental illnesses.

They look so clean – the tailored suit, sombre tie and jewelled pin,
The starched uniform and cap, gaily adorned with ribbons –
But their eyes are hard, dull and shifty, and imposing postures,
Incessant glances at the clock, give clues to corruption working within.

Is greed his motive force, trapped by the lust for power it buys?
Do status and recognition rule her latent lack of self-confidence?
Was childhood so devoid of love that clinical training
Could erode their inherent fellow feeling and humanity?

But my mind wanders, as I sit in pyjamas too big for me,
A borrowed dressing-gown – why am I here, did someone die

Mental Survival

Who was important to me? And, too late, their diagnosis is complete,
I realise that for them grieving is a disease, and I'm filled with pity.

How can I explain a lifetime of complex interactions in ten minutes?
My survival urge is weak, sapped by days of institutional food
And rules, and like a caged zoo animal, I placidly accept
This week's tortured care of experimental drugs and brainwashing ECT.

Oliver Swingler
25th October 2000

Oliver Swingler

Laughing

Laughed at, I shrink
And slink away,
Licking my wounds,
And pitying their ignorance
Ready wrapped in a clever act,
Dry minds devoid of feeling;
I want to ask if being mocked
Is beyond their experience,
Or are they seeking revenge
On someone weaker than
Whoever tormented them,
But fear and empathy
Tie my tongue,
Because I know they know,
And have no wish
To pierce an empty shell
And suffer reactive anger
Or imploding depression
I've caused,
Knowing I used to make fun of.
And maybe, possibly, perhaps,
Without my prompting,
Their life
Will eventually teach them
Lessons I've learned.

Laughed with, at myself,
I expand,
Parading my scars
Honourably won
In the struggles of my life,
Mistakes made

Mental Survival

For the umpteenth time,
Silly habits programmed into
My read-only brain
That serve as blessed antidotes
To arrogance,
Ever reminding me
I'm not a God or superhero,
But only a unique and special
Human being
Like everyone else,
Scrabbling around on the surface
Of a small planet,
At my best when aware
And openly admitting to
My relative unimportance
In the scheme of things
And many shortcomings.

Oliver Swingler
22nd October 2000

Oliver Swingler

Here's another poem I wrote to try to help my healing process ...
(sorry if some of the last verse does not make much sense outside the UK?)

In the ward

In the ward it was discovered
That every single one of us
Had been sexually, physically or emotionally abused
As a child,
Victims or a dictatorship,
Ruled by the older and stronger
Who sheltered behind the name of
Family values

They told us that our honest sensitivity
Being unable to pretend
That unwanted sex and violence
Made us happy,
And our difficulty in liking
Let alone loving
Those who caused us pain
Was unacceptable in a Christian society
And a weakness
That needed to be cured
With drugs and ECT
And by locking away

Then came 'community care'
And they put us in slum houses
In down-trodden districts
Surrounded by other vulnerable people
Whose lifestyles born of poverty and ignorance

Mental Survival

Were a constant reminder
Of what we had suffered,
And their newspapers called us mad, bad and dangerous
Saying we were the ones
Who did those crimes
Against humanity.

Victims once, victims twice, victims thrice.
Silent and lonely, alienated, depressed,
Desperately hoping the meek shall inherit the earth.

But the worm is turning,
Our suffering and trauma turns to strength and wisdom,
A self-respect for having survived their tortures,
Neither corrupted by hypocrisy, greed or power,
Nor losing our loving empathy
For nature and humankind –
Our plaintive whispers grow
As we encourage each other in tiny steps
And become magnified, an outraged chorus
Which will be heard;
We are many,
We have little to lose,
And nowhere else to go.

Oliver Swingler
4th November 2000
Amended 25.5.2916

Here's my third anti-ECT/anti-psychiatry poem, an acrostic poem (ie. all the first letters of the lines spell out …

ELECTRO-CONVULSIVE THERAPY

Elephants don't arrange to have memories wiped out
Larks don't sing tunes that awaken chronic doubt
Electric eels don't give shocks to others of their kind
Cheetahs don't advise speedy cures that damage the mind
Tortoises don't punish those who are a bit slower
Reindeer don't stigmatise whatever they see as lower
Owls don't manufacture darkness for hunting their prey
Crocodiles don't submerge animals in terror for pay
Oysters don't clam up if treatment is put to the test
Nightingales don't wilfully disturb other creatures' rest
Voles don't produce the dependence on hibernation
Unicorns don't pretend what's real is an invention
Locusts don't strip bare while announcing that it's healing
Spiders don't weave to confuse other spiders' feeling
Iguana don't make ugly innocent hope and belief
Vultures don't pick at the bones of those suffering grief

Mental Survival

Earthworms don't aim to undermine the vulnerable naïve
Tigers don't lurk behind caring postures that deceive
Hornets don't sting to sell results in published research
Eagles don't use old, weak ones to establish their perch
Rattlesnakes don't have hidden agendas that cause fear
Ants don't build nests that alienate every ant near
Psychiatrists and their drugs often do – they've done it to me
Yours may be the next mind to be raped by ECT

Oliver Swingler
October 2000

Oliver Swingler

My label

In my 55 years with the mentally ill label
My life has had its ups and downs, not entirely stable,
But one lasting received truth got printed on my brain
Implicit in every session, no need to explain
Why I was there, the whole focus of psychiatry
Said that I am the problem, yes the problem is me.

Was undermining my self-respect a conscious aim
Even before its birth, pointing the finger of blame,
Burdening a teenage child with overwhelming guilt
At being bad, rotten, dirty, diseased, perhaps built
From defective genes, amongst the crowd an alien,
Not much above a worm, an outcast mammalian?

So instead of helping, they ensnared and froze my mind
In victimhood, reinforcing my behaviour, blind
To the fact that both my parents had suffered child rape,
A childhood of sibling bullying with no escape,
An expectation of being treated much like dirt
A pattern established of mental trauma and hurt.

Yet I've never murdered, shot or knifed, tortured, blackmailed,
Sold into slavery, caused creatures wilful pain, gaoled
For fraudulently obtaining pensions from the old,
Nor caused economic crises in my lust for gold,
Beaten a partner or tried coercive control, spurned

Mental Survival

Climate change warnings in a dash for profits
unearned.

So who is more mentally ill, us or them, those who
Bear the stigma, the lowest of the low, yet are true
To themselves and strive to help others learn and
flower,
Or the rich, using divide and rule to cling to power,
Exporting bitter hatred to mask their own despair
In lives emptying of empathy and love and care.

Oliver Swingler
20th June 2016

Oliver Swingler

With love

The love of a mother, father,
By blood or adoptive,
Can fill the child
With self-worth
That lasts a lifetime
And confidence to meet the world
As an equal.

But inside the child of an abusive family,
Dysfunctional,
Is an empty feeling
Of lonely nothingness
A desperate yearning,
Searching to fill the void.

Perhaps wearing the mask
Of a salesperson
Or politician,
Or seeking fame,
The recognition of millions
On the stage
Or writing a book, a play, a poem
Like this one.

But it is a usually a vain quest
For never enough
Mostly attracting sycophants
And the also needy
A continuation of the lies,
The divorce
Between private and public life.

For there is no substitute.

Mental Survival

The hole can only be filled
With love.
Oliver Swingler
Not today Mr Death

What is happening to me? Who cares?
A day to day survival existence
Responding to letter, calls, conversations,
Mostly things that have upset or angered me,
Increasing the irritation of constant physical pain,
Nagging reminders of my dire past and shames,
A grind ing down periodof problems and negativity
–
No wonder I'm alone ...
And how long can I keep going, clutching at
The straws of books I've read before,
The daily crossword puzzle, incessant games
Of patience to fill my loneliness
And distract me from my abject misery ...

Totally reliant on the precious few
Moments of insight, warmth and inspiration,
Buoyant confirmations that my mind and ideas
Can still touch and help another
To do, be, think for themselves and grow,
Witnessing the beauty of empathy and love
Revealed in an act, look., word or gesture,
All crucial food for a stubborn belief that
Within the corrupt and hypocritical world
Which abused me
Within the certainty that I'm not the saviour
For people who can only be
The answer to their own predicaments,
There are enough sparks of humanity
Smouldering and building in readiness

Oliver Swingler

For the collapse of a greed driven economy
To nurture the traumatic transition to
The conscious coming of age of humankind,
Founded on the knowledge that we are not
The masters, the pinnacle of an evolutionary process
Which can do whatever the fuck it likes
And get away with it – as I used to think
In my childhood, adolescence and youth,
But a part of an integrated spirit, body, mind and feelings
In symbiotic relationship with the planet and universe
Which is so much more intelligent than out collective selves,
And maybe I'm still needed here, to learn and teach
By my own self-searching attitude of defiance
To both the domineering culture and victim mentality,
My allowing understanding of my current set of
Weaknesses, mistakes and failures –
So not today Mr Death
Maybe I'll put off
The alluring peace that beckons
For yet another stretch of time
And accept my proven ignorance of the future,
Surrender to the poignant power of healing hope,
And settle to living my life
Moment by moment, day by day.

Mental Survival

Know thyself

The ancients said,
According to a book I read,
'KNOW THYSELF' (and perhaps some understanding too
Would be a good idea) – and of course I do –
I've known me for 18,865.13 days,
Let alone the pre-birth phase,
I've known me as an obedient child,
Then in adolescence running wild,
And as an adult, parenting; I've known me
In more than 30 different jobs, as an employee
And as a boss, then made redundant, unemployed;
Sometimes a magnetic person, then someone to avoid;
Either joining in socially, or out of touch;
Part of a loving couple, or very much
Alone; full of life, or near death, and grieving;
Connected to the stars, or hopeless, unbelieving;
Drunk and sober; inspired, depressed;
At my worst and very best;
Being a fool, and wise; in credit and a debtor –
Yes I know me, and no-one knows me better!
But I must confess, that although I've made a long-term study
Of human biology, my knowledge is patchy, and my understanding muddy;
And efforts to record the cycles of my feelings have always lacked
The certainty to predict my next up or down as a fact;
And my numerous researches into psychology have yet to make clear

Oliver Swingler

Where my thoughts come from, and why the next good one should appear;
And as for my spirit – despite making countless lists
Of when it's filled me – I can't even prove that it exists!
And scientists have said,
According to another book I read,
After centuries of analysis, experiment and observation
Of all its forms in nature, and used in irrigation,
That they don't understand water – its workings are a mystery
To all of them – as they are to me,
Yet water, they are all agreeing,
Is over 70% of a human being,
By far the greatest part!
Oh dear, maybe I need to start
Again, first of all admitting, to tell
The truth, I don't know myself very well,
But this time, I've decided, only dying
Will make me give up trying.

Oliver Swingler
January 2000

Mental Survival

Love thy neighbour

The message 'Love thy neighbour as thyself' does not tell me to put other people first,
It rather counsels me build on and share my earned self-respect for my being and humanity,
For if I don't love myself, loving my neighbour is at best a pious aim, and more often an illusion or hypocrisy, an empty act of the moment,
Which may include a wish to be known as a 'loving person', a desire for special favours, a dream that someone else will be the answer to my own problems,
But if I can love my spirit even when it has been totally dormant and left me flat for weeks except for bursts of exhausting anger, and warming enthusiasm is a distant memory;
If I can love my body even when it is incapable of looking or doing what I want, and answers my every demand with complaint or illness, and only gives me worries which I've got enough of already;
If I can love my mind even when it fills my head with stupid nonsense which makes me seem a fool, or sniping judgmental criticism, or indecision and scatters every time I try to focus it;
If I can love my feelings even when they flood me with depression, and every experience confirms my doom and gloom, and death appears to be a welcome relief from my pain and suffering;
And still know that my spirit, body, mind and feelings are working for me, always doing their best, trying to give me the signals I need to be conscious of my current situation, and past, and what to do next, in their love of me,
Then loving my neighbour i s easy,

Oliver Swingler

And even if I don't believe that God or the universe or my neighbours love me, I know that something someone does,
And the rest happens naturally, it comes from a fullness that overflows, a wanting for the best, a recognition of the worth, an appreciation, of the struggles, and an empathetic love that has fewer and fewer conditions.

Oliver Swingler

Mental Survival

What a pity!

What a pity so many people seeking a spiritual path succumb to ideas that denigrate their physical home. The view that the spirit is good and the body bad, which can only result in a divided self, internal strife, a civil war with weapons of guilt and shame about natural functions, and an aim of unobtainable perfection in the pursuit of which there can only be losers.
The human body, my body is for me a glittering ray of illumination, an anchorage in reality, a university of enlightenment, and a daily source of wonder…

The head is a prime example of good leadership and management, constantly collecting information from within and outside via the nerves and five senses, a seasoned decision maker from its assessments and it also champions honesty, mostly going naked into the world with if nothing else the eyes never lying…

Support without demand for recognition of what is important is a quality that belongs with the neck and the throat teaches the necessity of being clear, of checking for and resolving promptly any blockages in relationships so that the carriers of life sustaining energy can pass without worry, unimpeded…

The arms and hands are an antidote to boredom, with their love of versatility – pointing the way and beckoning, admonishing and caressing, quick to improve upon their skills of touch and holding and their uninhibited playfulness makes me aware of my inner child, eager for expression…

Humility and care reside with the breasts in their potential function, when they totally focus on the survival needs of something else, working to become redundant, and they show in their requirement for security and extra vitamins and minerals that carers cannot long perform without looking after themselves.

The heart sets a standard of reliability, striving to adjust and give its best to running or walking or sleeping and its concerned involvement with its whole territory, the passion and drama it throws into every beat, the rest periods between bouts of great activity are all role models for my own behaviour…

Cleanliness and refinement are lessons from the intestines, open and braced to process through without undue complaint whatever comes next to them, sifting and sorting and extracting what is useful from food and experience and moving on and finally rejecting that which is out of date and could poison by its retention…

The waist gives a view of separation, above and below – not better or worse, all needed just different in its function and place. It can be an index of flexibility sometimes allowing a bending over backwards to achieve a harmony, whilst mindful of maintaining balance and its inner integrity…

Mental Survival

The possibility of regeneration is founded in the sex organs, nurturing the seeds to new life, as is the art of giving and receiving a joyful, warming pleasure. They embody a value for privacy and warn that what can heal can also hurt that power used without limit eventually corrupts including itself…

The hips and thighs seem to have an unbridled enthusiasm for free movement, once they get going the vigour is almost self-perpetuating and by their size and breadth and willingness to endure they remind me to try to broaden my scope and tolerate with relaxed ease the demands of reaching a goal…

Will drives the knees, intent on their forward aim, capped ready to protect against falls or short-term, absorbing the shocks that would incapacitate the less able, and by their complexity they promote the principle of specialisation, each part an expert in the together purpose of advancing the whole…

The ankles perhaps also give instruction or later life – they bear the weight of the entire body, and speak to me of taking my share of responsibility for everything I have joined and am part of and they also make me conscious of the advantages of farsightedness, to beware of impulsive acts that sprain or strain…

Does love enliven the feet, they take you and me where we want to go, in an all accepting empathy with an external command, an eternal optimism.

Oliver Swingler

They ground with mother earth, and by their connectedness unseen to the totality of the body, lend credence to the mysteries of life, the unknown universe beyond...

My spirit lives in my body and I don't believe that it is an obnoxious guest, always carping and criticising. I think it loves and values its home and listens to and learns from it and if I am on a spiritual path, maybe that's what I need to do too.
Oliver Swingler
4th December 1999

Mental Survival

Edited version of an article published by Dateline Magazine in March 2001

(Please don't take this as some sort of definitive relationship bible – or you're likely not to start any! Personally, I think there is no such thing as a perfect relationship, that all human beings are capable of getting on with all others, and that all relationships need to be worked at. That said, a good start helps, and these might be things you'd like to consider – and even discuss with a potential partner … And please note that I'm a hetero man – you can hopefully substitute she/him where you want)

Ask yourself. Is this the one?

Do I fancy her? Is there a spark of attraction lit by her spirit, form, voice or style that focuses me singularly, glad to watch myself strut flirtatiously, wanting to display my honest best, to initiate or promote courtship, forgetful of all else during and after our first encounter?

Does she fancy me? Is there in eye and smile and speech and posture some recognition and appreciation of my qualities, enough to offset the practical difficulties of a beginning? Is there real evidence in the nature of my welcome that here is where my love may take root and grow?

Can we readily discover many things in common? Does the conversation flow or flounder? Is there ease of playful banter or are jokes not understood even when explained? Are thoughts censored in fraught pauses, or does the speaking of one mind activate, enliven, open the other?

Do I feel safe with her and she with me? Are feelings, hurts and tears allowed, or do responses to them cause retreat behind a shell or act? Is there humility and care so that occasional bouts of moodiness are accommodated and not reacted to as the whole story?

Is she free? Distanced from the last so that it isn't a total rebound?   Is she looking for an important relationship with a man, rather than a woman, or wanting time to herself, or favouring one or more light liaisons? Does she have the confidence to face the world with whatever happens between us?

Are habits compatible? So that smoking or not, mannerisms of speech, irritations or criticisms said or unspoken don't block decent dealing? Is there concern about the health and welfare of the other, without one-sided dumping of problems, or the imposition of standards not freely agreed?

Is there harmony between us? Experienced in various circumstances – a meal, film, the pub, a walk in the country, meeting friends, relations, work colleagues? And when disagreements occur, is there sufficient will to listen and seek a compromise, rather than arguing from extreme entrenched positions?

Mental Survival

Is there deep engagement? Do revelations of past worsts shock or draw matching truth? Is sex a loving warming pleasure or do inhibitions or power trips leave either feeling used? Is a sometimes need for privacy respected? Have each worked through proving life crises, to be able to make a commitment?

Are our attitudes similarish? Is talking about them inspiring, learning and fun, or does discussion of race, politics, gender, religion, money, the environment produce anger or reticence building no-go areas? Is there tolerant desire for growth and change of the relationship and each within it?

Do our lives move in the same or parallel directions? Or are long-term plans or perceived purposes mutually exclusive? Is there room for a joint partnership to evolve or at least an attitude of protective support, content to watch and wait and will the other to greater wisdom and accomplishment?

Can I be myself with her and she with me? Is individuality nurtured? Is there acceptance of each as is now, or are exchanges driven by a vision of some future potential? Is each permitted separate friends and interests that don't threaten but rather strengthen the wanting to be together?

Are there conforming clues? Coincidences, reactions from strangers, indications from astrology, a feeling that this was meant to happen? Does romance flourish with flowers and poetry, beyond the myth of 'happily ever after' to a dedicated knowing that this is something worth working for?

Oliver Swingler

Mental Survival

Alas MAXIMUS   (to the tune of Greensleeves)

1   Oh MAXIMUS you do me wrong,
To treat me so robotically,
I was down and out, they stopped my dole,
I'm sick and homeless, in poverty.

(Chorus)   MAXIMUS said they really care,
When stats are all they want for their boss,
MAXIMUS said they're truly fair,
When all that concerns them is profit and loss.

2   They called me in for an interview
Where two flights of stairs blocked my wheelchair
MAXIMUS said I was fit for work
It's all my fault I couldn't get there

3   My doctors said that grief and abuse
Had caused me to become depressed
MAXIMUS said I was fit for work
As long as sometimes I could get dressed.

Chorus

4   I showed them my appointment card
For last-ditch chemotherapy
MAXIMUS said I was fit for work
If before I died I could bend my knee

5   But my friend witnessed the interview
And there's a tape which will reveal
MAXIMUS isn't fit for work
In evidence ready for my appeal

Oliver Swingler

Lyrics by Oliver Swingler and Making Waves Community Choir, version 1.2
Based in Cullercoats, near Newcastle

And on YouTube:
https://youtu.be/Hffu44-G9ZY

Mental Survival

Despairing NHS (to the tune of Clementine)

You might enjoy a song about privatisation
'Despairing NHS' – can it be saved?
http://youtu.be/MQ_EQ1koYEM

1.　　In the darkness, six feet under,
Bevan turning in his grave
Sixty-five years of free healing,
The NHS he cannot save.

Chorus:　　Oh our caring, oh our sharing,
Now despairing NHS,
Are you lost and gone for profit,
Privatised to serve the rich?

2.　　All the doctors, and the nurses,
Cleaners, porters do their best,
But their efforts no longer valued
In the growing profits quest.

3.　　Drug companies pay for research
And they promise us a cure
But all they want is extra profit
And to hell with the sick and poor.

Chorus

4.　　Clegg and Cameron keen to finish
Dismantling done by Brown and Blair,
PFI debts, target culture.
Reorganised for millionaires.

5.　　Shipman, Savile, Stafford hospital,
Just how bad can scandals get,

Oliver Swingler

Whistle-blowers, enquiries ignored,
But you ain't seen nothing yet!

Lyrics by Oliver Swingler & Making Waves choir, Cullercoats
Original Oh my darling Clementine: traditional
Version 2.2 August 2013

Mental Survival

Global Warming Song
(to the tune of 'What can we do with the drunken sailor?')

Chorus: What can we do about global warming?
What can we do about global warming?
What can we do about global warming?
Shrink our carbon footprint!

1. Walk, cycle, bus and train
Car share, avoid the plane
Holiday at home, learn to love the rain
Shrink our carbon footprint!

2. Insulate homes and get them lined
Stop oil, gas and coal being mined
Use tidal, solar, wind and find we'll
Shrink our carbon footprint!

Chorus: What can we do about global warming?
What can we do about global warming?
What can we do about global warming?
Shrink our carbon footprint!

3. Organic, local, seasonal eating
Recycle, mend, turn down the heating
Share, cooperate, stop competing
Shrink our carbon footprint!

Watch out! The seas are rising
Cry out! The seas are rising
Bale out! The seas are rising
Save our lovely planet!

4. Don't believe the greenwash, keep on prying
Tax millionaires, stop envy buying
Climate change deniers, they're all lying
Shrink our carbon footprint!

Chorus:
We can do a lot about global warming
We can do a lot about global warming
We can do a lot about global warming
Save our lovely planet!

Lyrics by Oliver Swingler and Making Waves choir, Cullercoats, UK – Version 3 March 2013"
Making Waves choir singing the song on YouTube: http://youtu.be/s9g_Ucr4twQ

Mental Survival

Bees song
(To the tune of All Through The Night)

Bees are buzzing, pollinating
All through the day
Feeding larvae, honey making
All through the day
But we make their lives confusing
Neonicotinoids using
They get ill, our crops we're losing
All through the day

Wild insects pollen blending
All through the day
So that plants can be unending
All through the day
But monoculture ploughs are slashing
It's their habitats we're trashing
And their numbers they are crashing
All through the day

Promote wildlife gardens growing
All through the day
Stop the GM farmers sowing
All through the day
Help the bees to keep maturing
Harmful chemicals outlawing
Farms organic need restoring
All through the day

Version 2.1 – Lyrics by Oliver Swingler and Making Waves choir, Cullercoats, UK
https://youtu.be/TwHZkY4UbfI

Oliver Swingler

Lily Matthews Fund

My mother Lily Matthews – known to us as Anne Swingler – was born in Shieldfield, Newcastle, a notorious slum district, in 1915. Her father was illegitimate – causing a schism as her mother's family hadn't wanted the marriage to go ahead – and he was probably already in the First World War trenches (and possibly already shell-shocked) when Lily was born. At the end of the war, there being no work, and the family schism, they moved to London – but in 1923 her mother died of TB, and then some 4 years later her father raped her. There she was, in a strange city, bullied because of her accent, horribly abused by the only person she thought she could trust. And there was no support available – a girl reporting being raped was liable to locked away in an asylum for life.

In 1987 when she was 73, I was the first person Annie told of her trauma. She spoke to family members, a few close friends, but after a week or so didn't want it mentioned again – it was just too painful. Meanwhile we'd worked out that my father Stephen was also raped whilst a pupil at public school.

For me it explained so much, the loveless childhood in a dysfunctional family – some years later I had some counselling, and found that my psychology was similar to someone who had themselves been sexually abused, even though I wasn't. But in a sense it was also for me too late.

Mental Survival

Such was the sibling rivalry I was born into, that during my childhood, my sister twice did things that could have resulted in my death, and she'd wind our elder brother up to attack me – I used to wet the bed, hide under it, have nightmares, stammer, blush – all the symptoms of abuse. At 12/13 I was stealing, smoking, drinking and bunking off school, sent to a psychiatrist and given a load of Freudian bullshit – then in 1971, after my finals and grieving the death of my father my mother and sister got me sectioned, where I was given ECT. Three years later, I was involved in an 'incident' with the police, convicted of assaulting 3 officers (1 true!), badly beaten up, spent a few weeks in prison getting out on appeal, and then almost killed myself. After a year recovering in a Richmond Fellowship hostel, I realised I couldn't cope on my own, and was a sucker for recruitment by my sister into an esoteric cult, remaining a member for 19 years.

But there was another family thread in that my father and mother met in the 1930s whilst members of the Communist Party, Stephen after the war becoming left Old Labour MP for Stafford (later Newcastle-under-Lyme), and a junior minister in the Wilson government, and our upbringing also involved CND Aldermaston marches, Anti-Apartheid and Young Socialists. In the 1964 election I was running the committee rooms in my father's constituency, canvassing in run-down pottery and mining villages, asking people to vote for my father their socialist candidate – and after he was elected with a thumping majority, we returned to our very comfortable home in Hampstead. The contradiction was obvious to me, and after doing a year's VSO, at college I joined the International Socialists, was Chairman of the Socialist Society the year we had a sit-in, and later was a NUPE Shop Steward, and more recently have been chair of a user-run mental health co-operative, and of more than one tenants and residents association. Although whilst a member of the cult I was a yuppie in the 1980s – government sales manager of a computer company – I never quite lost my beliefs.

When I researched the family tree, I found that one ancestor was a Colonel in the Indian Army, at a time when natives were shot without trial, another a part owner of an ironworks in Derbyshire which undoubtedly used child labour, and there were large investments in South American railways, which were built using slave labour.

I told my mother many years ago that I didn't want any inheritance, because not only as a socialist do I not believe in property ownership, but also I regard the inheritance as dirty money. And think the conspicuous consumption invariably exhibited by the very rich in a world of finite and diminishing resources – of water, food, raw materials, fuel, accelerating over-population, and global warming – is utterly unsustainable, a mental illness of greed, making the problems in a period of economic crisis completely insoluble.
However she chose not to believe me. So when my mother died, I had a Deed of Variation written

Mental Survival

to her will, whereby after some going to my son, for an astrology research project, and to pay for my funeral, the bulk went to the Community Foundation as the Lily Matthews Fund. From which I've tried in a small way to rectify the balance, to try to break the cycle of abuse, by using the money to support charities to do with my mother's and my life – such as Tyneside Rape Crisis Centre, and Someone Cares – and also environmental groups, including Friends of the Earth, and Marie Stopes International, and especially local projects in the fields of women's and green issues – that it may counter some of the worst aspects of my family history, and where the money came from.

Oliver Swingler

Oliver Swingler

Psychiatric drugs and the diagnosis lottery
(Important: Before even thinking about coming off them, please read the note at the bottom)

I've had a number of different psycho labels, whose only real use was allowing me to access talking therapies which I desperately needed, and get on the benefit register so I wouldn't starve whilst having a period of respite from the job market, which I was temporarily unable to cope with. And I've known quite a few people who have 'earned' more than one utterly contradictory diagnosis depending on which psychiatrist sat and observed them for 10 minutes to half an hour!

But this often totally arbitrary diagnosis can be crucial, not least because each flavour - which can follow a person around for the rest of their life - leads to a completely different set of behaviour-affecting psycho drugs each with its particular set of side-effects.

And for better or worse many people on psycho drugs didn't get beyond their GP (who've probably forgotten most of their brief mental health lectures), who certainly didn't have half-an-hour to listen to a patients often difficult to articulate symptoms, and are all too ready to believe the advertising blurb in medical journals or glib promises trotted out by commission-only drug company reps extolling the latest wonder drug!

There've been umpteen scandals associated with psychiatric drug – such that only 13% of

Mental Survival

Americans believe that pharmaceutical companies are "generally honest and trustworthy," – Valium with its highly addictive properties, Prozac, Seroquel, Ritalin; the list is endless. Authors of supposedly independent research papers have been found to have financial ties to manufacturers, while negative results, even deaths, in drug trials have been hidden away beyond public view until a court case forced out the truth – too late for many – and whistleblowers hounded out of the profession to protect exorbitant drug company profits.

Some years ago I knew a lovely woman, and we really hit off. She'd lived with the label manic–depressive for years, and was utterly dependent on lithium. I hadn't seen her for a bit, and then she rang, we met up, and she told me of feeling progressively more unwell, visit to the doctor and tests, and being told the lithium was killing her, her kidneys and thyroid were too damaged , she didn't have long –and she died a few weeks later. And, I've known people who had a fairly mild depressive episode, prescribed a psycho-drug, and within a week committed suicide.

Psycho drugs are dangerous, psycho drugs can kill – and I'd advise anybody – do your damnedest not to get on them in the first place.

IMPORTANT NOTE
Yes, psycho drugs are dangerous, but coming off them can be even more dangerous. Many have highly addictive properties (which is maybe why the drug companies make such huge profits!?)

and a sudden cessation can cause drastic mood swings, violent episodes and acute suicidal tendencies.

What's usually needed is a gradual weaning off process with at a minimum some sort of supportive network of family, friends, maybe holistic healers who can spot the signs of how withdrawal is affecting you, and preferably as the long-term loving care of a supportive community. I'm totally aware that is simply not available to the vast majority of people –and at current levels of mental health funding, unlikely ever to be so. Perhaps that should be a focus of our campaigning?

Mental Survival

3 experiences of mental health stigma:

Firstly, after I was sectioned and given ECT in 1972, I tried vainly to get a job, making the mistake of being honest about where I'd been the last 3 months – and didn't get a single reply to my letters, let alone a interview. So I concocted a CV with completely false bits, including one of the references a fictitious person at an address a friends could pick up, for me to write myself! I soon learnt to only apply for jobs which weren't too fussy, businesses where what was important was proving in the first month you could do it rather than history –and had little trouble getting jobs between periods of unemployment and crisis!

But in 1989 I applied for a job in the charity sector, and declared my whole mental health history, arguing that because of not despite my experience I'd developed a store of empathy for a whole range of people and could better do the role (as a volunteer co-ordinator). I got an interview, but didn't get either of the 2 jobs – but a couple of weeks later, a phone-call and, someone had dropped out, was I interested - you bet, and I was with CSV for 5 years!

Secondly, I was once with my GP when he suddenly started talking about 'mad people' this and 'mad people that, whilst giving me sly looks to see how I was reacting. I didn't, but immediately after the session went to the local advocacy project to help me lodge a formal complaint, which went through a Health Authority mediator – who believed me not them, and the GP and Practice manager were both forced to apologise. (But they got their own back – a large chunk of my medical records had gone missing!

Thirdly, over the years I've joined a number of on-line dating sites (even at 68 I haven't given up hope!), and met some really nice women. I don't want to shock, but I do like to be honest, particularly as being an ECT-survivor still affects my memory, mood swings etc. So at some point in the conversation when we're exchanging history I'll mention mental health. – and get one of 3 main responses: either, she'll freeze, the conversation will abruptly end however well we were getting on previously, and she'll find some excuse to high-tail it out of there (perhaps after having a go at me for not mentioning it on my profile); or she'll be incredibly sympathetic on the surface, but I can sense the chances of any relationship developing have reduced to zero – I'm high risk (!); or, my revelation will draw out her own, and we'll have a much deeper conversation without any judgment on either side.

Mental Survival

Sometimes it pays to be known as a trouble-maker

For years I carried this victim mentality around, bullied by siblings, put through the mental health system and ECT, expelled from school, in prison (at least in part) for things I didn't do – until one month I got assaulted on 3 separate occasions by youths. I decided I wouldn't put up with it any more, being treated without dignity and respect, and with the help of Victim Support, complained to the police and head-teachers, and felt so much better in myself for having taken a stance.

I then went further, and with the help of advocates, pushed through a complaint against a doctor who'd started talking about 'mad people' during my consultation, and eventually wrung an apology from him and the Practice Manager via the Heath Authority conciliator (who believed me, not them).

On another occasion my benefit was stopped for no good reason, which caused my mental health to take a nose-dive. But instead of just stuming and getting more depressed to the point of suicidal, I turned my anger outwards, and managed to get a solicitor via the local Law Centre, and eventually not only got all my backdated money owed, but also an extra payment of 100 quid as compensation for harassment or whatever they called it.

Soon after Atos got the DWP contract, I got a letter calling me in for an interview – six months before my 65th birthday. So I immediately replied saying I'd be glad to attend, and oh, I'd be coming with my advocate, who'd be tape-recording the whole interview. A week before the interview, Atos sent me another letter saying they'd had a further look at my medical notes, no need to attend for interview, my benefits would continue, as far as I can remember, for my lifetime!

I don't know if this is unique – Atos backing off before a fight – but the only reason I can think of is that the DWP file on me at that time was so full of complaints – that they knew I'd take appeals the distance, to the European Court if necessary, and decided it just wasn't worth it.

I'm quite fortunate in that I tapped into some part of my character which not only revels in a struggle against authority, but also quite enjoys being known as a rebel or trouble-maker. But it can be exhausting and mentally draining, and I'd advise anyone, if you do decide to take this path – make sure you have good support systems in place, all the lovely people who are on your side, maybe family, friends, an advocate, CAB, solicitor – don't do it on your own – you'll need them!

Mental Survival

What psychiatrists, mental health workers and carers need to know about survivor/user groups

Mental health groups which are entirely survivor/user run are very different from those involving (and often managed by) psychiatrists, mental health workers and carers. The latter, however well intentioned, have a problem in that survivors who have experienced being sectioned by people they trusted – and then receiving psychiatric drugs and/or ECT with no consent let alone informed consent, and damaging after-effects which may last a lifetime – will naturally be extremely wary if not downright terrified of people who have the power to lock away.

So if psychiatrists etc are present at a meeting, survivors may be less than open and honest, say what they think the psychiatrist wants to hear, if not downright lie as an instinctive survival tactic. To the extent that the psychiatrist may even have diagnosed as borderline catatonic someone who happily chats away in the company of survivors who can deeply empathise with his or her state of mind and experiences – something I've actually witnessed, but the professional never did.

To illustrate, one of my encounters with psychiatry went like this:
Whilst exhausted and grieving the death of my father, I was sectioned by my mother and sister, given deep sleep therapy, and then when I didn't get 'well' quickly enough – it was a short-stay hospital – given ECT (and 45 years later I still

suffer after-effects of chronic daily memory problems, suicidal thoughts, mood swings). As far as I can recollect, and it is hazy, the psychiatrist saw me for about 5 minutes and didn't ask me a single direct question. Some weeks later I was desperate to get out of the clinic, and another patient suggested going to art therapy, and painting a picture using only bright colours signifying I was getting better, dark equalling depression! And it worked, the art therapist got very excited, this time I did have a conversation with the psychiatrist, lied through my teeth about how positive I felt, and was set free.

Since 1974 I have personally refused any care that involved psychiatrists, such has been my fear of their power, and disgust at past experience of the abuse of it.

How you get around that I don't know – but you need to factor in that it is quite likely what we're telling you may be a lot more positive, amenable and complimentary than we're thinking.

Some thoughts on violent crime and "mental illness"

https://www.facebook.com/oliver.swingler.9/posts/10210832715713188

All too often when an appalling crime of violence occurs without any seeming rhyme or reason, eventually the media will settle on the consensus that the perpetrator was "mentally ill", and that is supposed to explain it.

But not only does it explain very little, it also unfortunately leaves us easy targets, the considerable community of mental health survivors – whose only 'crime' may be to suffer chronic mental distress since being abused as children – with yet more isolation through increased pariah status stigma.

The often research confirmed fact needs repeating over and over again – that mental health survivors are far more likely to be victims of violence than perpetrators. Mental health survivors are far more likely to be victims of violence than perpetrators. And not only that, if we do become violent, it is far, far more likely that it will be turned in on ourselves with self-harm, cries for help and serious suicide attempts, than outwards.

And when 'mental illness' is linked to violence, all too often a causative link can be found to psychiatric drugs, with their long history of insufficient testing and cover up. Either those drugs produced side-effects sufficient to alter the character of the patient, or in desperation because of those side-effects, the patient stops taking the drugs, suddenly and without help, with the same consequences.

We live in a society of massive disparity of wealth, where greed, celebrity status and hypocrisy are rewarded, with the media ever eager to do the bidding of the rich and powerful promoting divide and rule, fostering suspicion and hatred – black against white, young old, women men, Christian Moslem, gay straight – whilst like-minded social media groupings tend to reinforce prejudices learnt at home and school. And at the same time there is massive pressure to conform, with instead of individuality being celebrated, vicious troll-like internet condemnation and abuse stamps on anyone who dares disagree with the herd, whilst hundreds of imaginary friends is considered more important than real best buddies – "Some of my best friends are ..." may not be proof of tolerance, but no best friends at all is a much better breeding ground for bigotry.

No wonder that so many particularly men – less able to articulate feelings that show weakness, more likely to be told, snap out of it, don't be such a wimp – should feel alienated from society and themselves. And if they do manage to get into the system, they then discover that a 10 minute diagnosis of complex life history and feelings labels them as the problem, the psychiatrist's dream of a rogue male probably with deficient genes, who also needs to be avoided for fear of contagion.

Mental Survival

All too often if someone does muster the courage to ask for help, they find themselves at the back of massive waiting list for talking therapies, disbelieved by the DWP and its privatised minions, stigmatised as the lowest of the low, lost in a chronically underfunded mental health system, the brunt of the worst hypocrisy as each successive government promises to prioritise mental health knowing that non-earmarked funding will be used by councils and health authorities for different populist priorities.

So when you next hear that a violent crime was committed by someone who was "mentally ill", don't blame us – look to your own prejudices, society at large, health priorities, profiteering drug companies, and the mass media and their millionaire masters who propagate the hatred that breeds alienation and violence, to deflect criticism from themselves.

Oliver Swingler
18th June 2016

Oliver Swingler

Pioneers of the Human Spirit

Recently I went to my first Lifeboat meeting (note Lifeboat was Tyneside Mental Health Cooperative, a totally user/survivor run group in Newcastle), and had this curious feeling of coming home. The meeting, the atmosphere, the people reminded me so much of my stay in a mental hospital and half-way house. What is it about mental health survivors that's different?

This is what I pondered, and here are some thoughts...
- there is often a much greater than average allowance and tolerance, and conversely much less judgment and expectation, so people can feel safe and be themselves, quirks, eccentricities, warts and all, without trying to be perfect, or something they are not, and nonetheless as equal as everyone else
- there tends to be a lot of sensitivity to surroundings and empathy for others, and sometimes a very deep listening, not just to what people are saying, but also to what they are not saying (which is vital, as some people express themselves best in many other ways than words) ..
- there can be a slowing of time, not so much frantic rushing about, much tea and chat, ready to wait for as long as it takes for another person to open up ..
- there can be a very high degree of personal honesty and self-knowledge, learned the

hard way, the wisdoms that come from hard knocks, having been tried and tested ..
- there's often much less importance given to external features (such as looks, fashion, class, accent) and more to inner human qualities like care and warmth.
-

And I was thinking, wouldn't I want the world to be like that?

Sometimes I've watched people, trapped in positions of power and wealth and fame, hooked by politics or yuppiedom, believing those things important, and wondered – who are the most mentally ill? What a life of pain and misery for the inner person, a loneliness, surrounded by hypocrisy, greed, and corruption, and fair-weather friends …

There's some special quality about those defined as being mentally ill, with or without choice refusing to play the game, that calls society to attention. In my own medical notes, I'm described as having a 'personality disorder' (amongst other things – I suspect a label earned as punishment for refusing to cooperate with psychiatry!) – this was given as weakness, but I now regard it also as a strength, that I was strong enough to defy the massive pressure to conform to rules and regulations that went against my natural feelings and instincts, and ways of behaviour that I knew to be stupid.

In times in history the 'mentally ill' have been cherished as being 'touched by god'. In many places the village 'fool' was looked after, and listened to for insights most unusual, and one even held a high position closest to the king. In some ancient tribes no-one was allowed to begin training as a venerated shaman or healer unless they had experienced some sort of life crisis or mental breakdown.

Pain is a natural signal, that says something is wrong – and so is mental pain and anguish, struggling with grief and depression, perhaps wrestling with regret at something done or not done, said or left unsaid. What a shame that society at large deals with it by overriding, with powerful drugs or ECT, rather than listening, to the inner cries of anguish, taking to heart whatever lessons can be learnt, to change, put thing right, seeking to heal the ills of society, instead of shooting the messenger, blaming and stigmatising the patient.

I've always found it curious that even in the New Age movement exhibitions have been called Mind, Body, Spirit – in our ultra rational world, missing out vital feelings. Yet it is just those feeling too strong to ignore that may first earn the mentally ill label, feelings that cast off the cloak of personality, of empathy for individuals and a group sensitivity, to what doesn't fit in the act of a psychiatrist or politician, feelings that give a lie to the supposed primary gene of self-interest, that want to help.

And there's another aspect – what is sometimes called the paranormal. Not so long ago, masses of mostly women were burnt as witches for seeing

Mental Survival

things, hearing voices, dealing in the inexplicable, and it does beg the question whether the denial of feeling is part of the same thread of misogyny running through mainstream treatment of mental health .. There are many complementary therapies, subjects like astrology, telepathy and clairvoyance, which defy proof, yet neither can they be disproven to scientific standards. As an ex-cult, I'm very aware how such subjects can attract charlatans, but surely the lack of understanding, of dark matter, the unused capacity of the humn brain, might at least recommend an open mind, and not to dismiss out of hand such groups as the Spiritual Crisis Network, which can see a crisis as likely signalling a pioneering breakthrough as a disease?

A couple of days ago I visited a closed Facebook site, on which someone had posted their heart-rending saga of abuse at the hands of psychiatry, forced drug treatment, the removal of all human choice and dignity, the humiliation of locking away, and all this in a supposed democratic country, a world leader in human rights. And what followed was an outpouring of support and love, empathy and counsel – member after member showing they cared, offering word of comfort, another way to look at it, things that had worked for them.

And I was thinking, wouldn't I want the world to be like that?

Oliver Swingler
24th June 2016

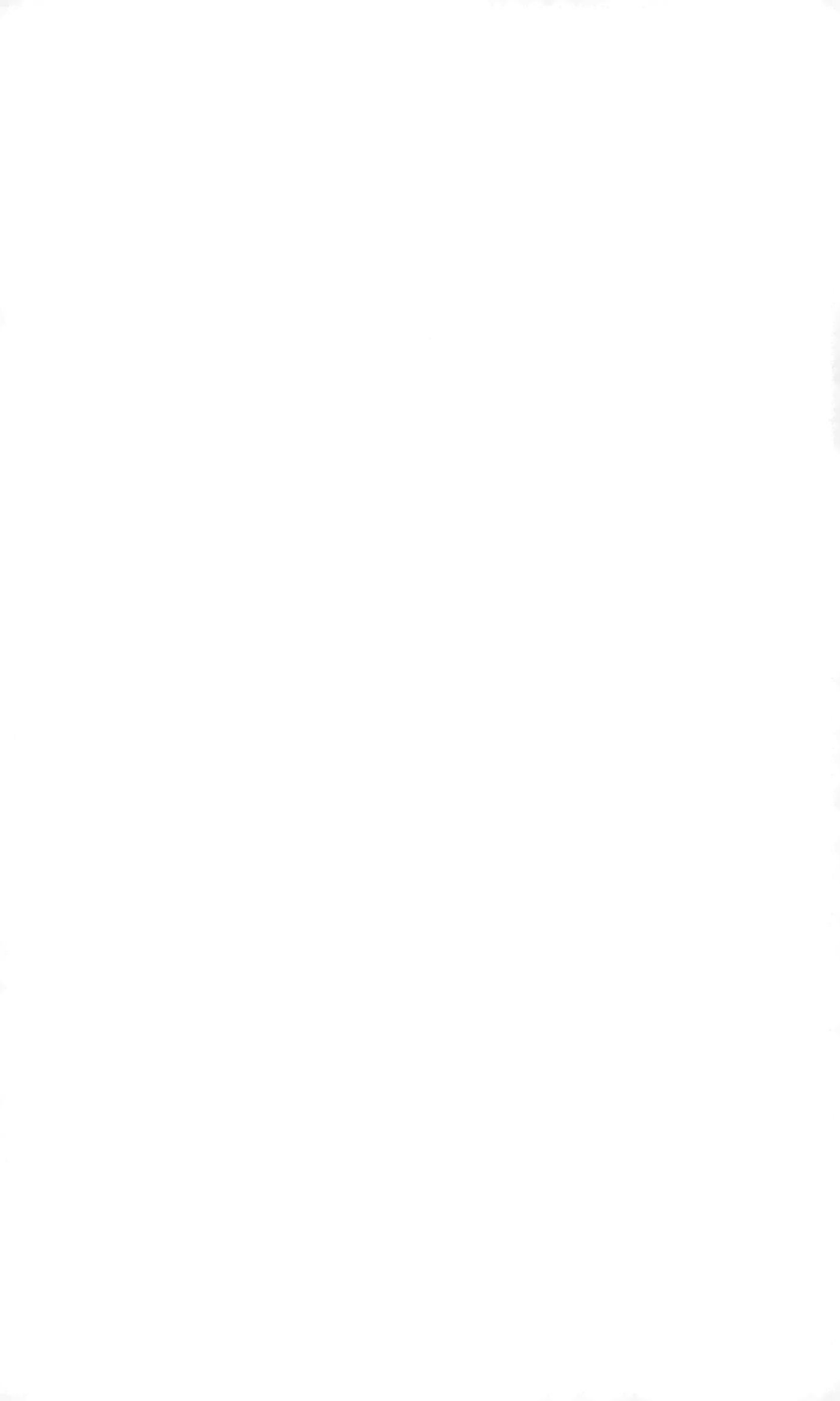

www.ingramcontent.com/pod-product-compliance
Ingram Content Group UK Ltd.
Pitfield, Milton Keynes, MK11 3LW, UK
UKHW041412180426
11947UKWH00007B/93